Dementia

The Monster Within

Dementia
The Monster Within

A Calm Before The Storm

*A Person's Journey through the Pitfalls of Dementia
and Our Medical System*

By

Karla Abel

Published by

Abel Publishing

Dedication

This book is dedicated to the hospice teams, my brother, Kevin Stoltz, my husband's nephew, Bryan and his wife Ruby Abel, and all the caregivers with loved ones dealing with this disease.

Table of Contents

Acknowledgements

I would like to give a personal thanks to all the wonderful people that helped and supported Ray and I throughout our journey with dementia. This includes the hospice teams, the doctors and nurses, Home Solutions, The Alzheimer's Association, High Ridge Fire Department, Help At Home employees, Aging Ahead, and the nursing homes that cared for Ray during the respite visits. I'd also like to thank my friends (Judy Strawhun, Ginger Johnson, Laura Norcutt), my brother, Kevin Stoltz, the members of Four Winds Garden Club, neighbors (Earl and Betsy), and of course, Ray's nephew and his wife, Bryan and Ruby Abel.

Introduction

Dementia takes a heavy toll on the caregivers; this includes finances, emotions, physical, and in losing the loved one. Dementia is a slow progressive disease that robs our loved ones of their personality, their dignity, their mind and reduces them to a helpless unresponsive state before death. The hardships the caregivers face while caring for their charges is unbelievable. They face a minefield of obstacles, including financial ruin due to the cost of care in the home and/or nursing homes, not knowing how to deal with the violence and personality changes, the patients wandering off, the emotional ups and downs, the physical toll on the caregiver and the lack of support from the community, family, friends, and governmental programs. Many caregivers have worked all their lives just to lose everything due to this horrible disease.

The REAL help is out there, but limited, and hard to find. There is plenty of information on help from nursing homes or home care if you have unlimited funds. To get Medicaid you must spend down the loved one's money until they only have their social security to pay for the nursing home room. I will discuss this further in the last chapter.

Chapter 1: Genetic Predisposition, Early Signs

Our journey with dementia often begins with contributing factors that include a list of health issues due, to unhealthy eating habits, lifestyle and genetics. My husband, Ray's dementia developed due to atherosclerosis, (hardening of the arteries) caused by high triglycerides, and cholesterol, which restricted blood flow to the entire body. Blood carries oxygen to the brain and if restricted, will cause damage. Unhealthy lifestyle practices can contribute to heart disease, diabetes, stroke and dementia. Unhealthy eating habits, smoking, drinking alcohol or soda can affect our health.

In addition, we have inherited traits that can cause some people to be affected sooner in life. Ray's dementia developed earlier than normal because of inherited traits. Ray's mother and older brother both had dementia. Ray also had two other brothers with cardiovascular issues. Studies have shown that we need to be mindful of what foods we are eating, and how much we are smoking and drinking so that we can live a healthier lifestyle.

Our story begins with Ray, eating poorly, smoking and drinking early in his life. I was able to influence him in mid-life to stop smoking, drinking and to start eating better. Unfortunately, it was not soon enough. He started showing concerning blood tests (extremely high levels of triglycerides numbers) early in his forties. He did not have a weight problem like many people with poor eating habits, nor diabetes, and had a near normal blood pressure. However, I was concerned that his triglycerides were so high as compared to my numbers, but his cholesterol was near normal. I discussed this with the doctor, it was noted, but not a concern at that time. Over time his blood vessels narrowed due to atherosclerosis all through his body.

On the Monday before Thanksgiving in 2006 at the age of 62 he had a heart attack. He was complaining of chest pain all day but thought it was indigestion. Later when I mentioned that he did not look good he admitted he did not feel good. I read the heart attack symptoms from a book on health which finally persuaded him to go to the emergency room. He did not want to acknowledge a problem and did not want to have to stay at the hospital.

I reassured him that we were just going to check out his heart and if it was ok, he would come home. However, he was admitted to the hospital for further tests and a cardiac catheterization showed a 100% closed right carotid artery and the left side 60% closed. He underwent and survived a quintuple bypass surgery and thankfully did not suffer a stroke or any other complications. The quintuple bypass is the most intricate heart bypass surgery and includes all five of the major arteries feeding the heart. With blood flow restricted to his brain, he was a good candidate for developing dementia and/or stroke.

Ray had retired from Chrysler in 2000 at the age of 56. I was still working at Monsanto. During this period (roughly from 2000 to 2014) we were not really aware that Ray had early dementia. I was dealing with health issues of my own after being diagnosis with cancer in 2007. I also lost my mother in 2007 and had surgeries in 2008 and 2013 to prevent my cancer from returning.

We owned 58 acres and boarded horses at our farm. I also broke and trained a horse for me to ride. I landscaped the grounds around the house and helped Ray finish building our house. I continued to work at Monsanto four more years after Ray retired but was laid off in 2004. I found a temporary job for a year and a half and was laid off again. I did not find another job so I decided to retire. In addition to boarding horses, I volunteered at the Missouri Botanical Garden, worked on the Floral Display for the Veiled Prophet Parades, and belonged to a garden club. Of course, when Ray began to advance in his disease, I had to work around his illness, but not give up my activities in order to keep my sanity.

The dementia disease process is defined through seven stages[1] which will be applied to Ray's symptoms in the chapters ahead. The Seven Stages of Dementia are:

- Stage 1 (No cognitive decline)
- Stage 2 (Very mild cognitive decline)
- Stage 3 (Mild cognitive decline)
- Stage 4 (Moderate cognitive decline)
- Stage 5 (Moderately severe cognitive decline)
- Stage 6 (Severe cognitive decline)
- Stage 7 (Very severe cognitive decline)

With this background of our situation, I will embark upon our journey to deal with Ray's *Dementia, The Monster Within.*

Chapter 2: The Beginnings of Confusion

Ray progressed through the first three stages of dementia from 2000 to 2005. At Stage One (No cognitive decline) the detection of the disease is very subtle. It is hard to tell if the person is just forgetful or if something is wrong. The person appears to not have any cognitive problems at this point. The narrowing of Ray's arteries continued and *Dementia, The Monster Within* was on its path to destruction.

After Ray retired from Chrysler in 2000 outwardly, he did not show any signs. He continued to take care of the horses and our farm. He finished the basement and the house. He kept his appointments as scheduled, cut the grass, and baled the hay as needed. In addition, he would go over to his favorite brother's house to help him work on his house. I was still working and everything seemed to be going fine; I didn't observe any changes. I handled the scheduling of appointments, financial matters, and other business and household management tasks.

At Stage Two (Very mild cognitive decline) from 2006 to 2009, after he had had his heart attack, he started to forget dates, appointments, where he left his tools, and how to do things. On days that he had an appointment I had to remind him several times of the time. Ray did the grocery shopping on Fridays for us. Once I retired in 2006, I went with him to the store and I noticed that he was having trouble making change.

He was becoming moody and was losing his ability to concentrate. This was most evident in his work on a specific piece of equipment, the hay baler. To use the hay baler, it is important to regulate the tension on the twine that makes the bales. Because Ray forgot how to set it up, he set the tension too tight and broke the knotters (the part that contains the needles where the twine is threaded to make the square bales). To replace it, he went to a sale and bought another baler just like the one he had broken. I did not know he had dementia and went along with his thought that something was wrong with the baler. If I had known he had cognitive issues we would have bought a different baler with better quality knotters and a different set up.

At Stage Three (mild cognitive decline) from 2010 to 2011, Ray was starting to forget more and more of what he was doing. He continued to have trouble baling the hay and again broke the knotters in this new baler. In 2010, we were setting up the new barn to board horses at our place and he seemed confused about how to build a tack room. He had constructed other projects just a couple of years earlier and was very familiar with laying out a wall, framing it and standing it in place. He forgot how to do it. I had to help him lay it out and put it together. He had to repeat taking measurements several times. He could not build it like he did before and was making several mistakes.

He had trouble installing electrical receptacles and switches, which he had done many times before. Also, he was having difficulty plumbing a new bathroom at his brother's house.

He said he was having trouble backing the car up and was getting too close to the wall so he placed tape on the garage floor to help him park the car. He was losing his depth perception. I did think it was strange, but dismissed it at the time. He started to repeat his sentences and his actions which I also thought was weird.

Chapter 3: Inability to Do Tasks

During Stage Four (Moderate cognitive decline) from 2011 to 2014, doctors continued to monitor Ray's atherosclerosis. His blood vessels continued to narrow and corresponded with worsening dementia symptoms. In the summer of 2011, Ray had a stent inserted in his left carotid artery. I also began to notice careless behavior from my usually always responsible and hardworking husband.

In February of 2013, I had a double mastectomy to prevent my 2007 cancer from coming back. Ray drove me to the hospital. After my surgery, I found that Ray had left the hospital. I called Ray and asked why he left and was not there when I woke up. Because he did not have a good answer, he stated that he was told to leave and not to come back. This was not true, of course. I was released the next day and had a friend drive me home.

When I arrived home, I noticed that Ray could no longer follow instructions or perform even simple tasks, like filling the buckets with water and placing them in the stalls for the horses, anymore. I had to do the chores and take care of the horses with my surgical drains still in place for a week. He also started doing strange things like destroying items that I wanted to keep (e.g. chopped up some railroad ties and an old wagon).

Another job he had proficiently done regularly was running electric fencing to keep the horses in the pasture. Rather than wrapping the wire once around a conductor, he would wrap the wire several times and forget to run the wire to the next conductor. He could not follow though and finish the task.

It seems that when you have horses you are continually setting up and repairing fencing. In the past, Ray had no problem installing fencing. About this time, I began to notice that Ray needed specific instructions on how to stand a fence pole in the ground and hammer it in place. Rather than running the wire perpendicular to the post so it could be clipped to the post, he incorrectly wrapped the wire around the fence post several times and did not follow through to the next post. I also had to be present to show him how to attach the clip that holds the wire to the post. He kept repeating the same mistakes over and over and could not seem to remember how to do it.

During Ray's 2013 annual wellness check, I mentioned to his primary care physician that he was having anger issues, repeating his actions, and was forgetful. The doctor suggested Ray may have dementia and prescribed Aricept to treat confusion related to Alzheimer's disease. Aricept is an enzyme blocker that works by restoring the balance of natural substances (neurotransmitters) in the brain and may improve memory, awareness, and the ability to function.[2]

We had to increase the dosage slowly and at lower doses it was working fine. However, when we got to the prescribed dose, he started having more anger issues; I kept him on the prescribed dosage for about two weeks expecting improvement until I could not deal with his violence anymore. I learned that anger is a side effect of the drug so I reduced the dosage over time until he was removed from the Aricept. His anger issues returned to the lower level it was before the use of Aricept.

During the next year's (2014) visit, I informed the doctor that I had taken Ray off the Aricept and noted that he had additional significant behavioral changes. I also mentioned to the doctor that Ray was having trouble using the TV remote control and washing the dishes. He was repeating his actions, and sentences, having mood changes, and depression. The doctor gave him the standard neurological evaluation test to see if he could draw a clock's hands. He failed and did not know the date, time, who the president was and other items.

About this time, Ray was starting to have driving issues and forgetting where places were located. He was not getting lost, but was getting confused. Because of this, I only let him drive when I was in the car, except for one time which was a costly mistake. His brother wanted Ray to go to the ballgame with him. I didn't want them to take the car because it was overheating and I wanted to take it to the dealer to check it out. They drove it anyway; it overheated, they towed the car home and missed the game. The motor was ruined and I had to get a new motor.

In June of 2014, following the doctor's recommendations, to prevent further driving issues and for Ray's safety, I took the keys from him and didn't allow him to drive at all. It was hard to do, but I blamed the doctor and Ray gave up the keys. Ray continued to try to drive so I hid the keys.

Chapter 4: Wandering

During Stage Five (Moderately severe cognitive decline) from 2015 to 2016, the primary care doctor recommended that Ray be evaluated by a neuropsychologist. I described Ray's symptoms to the doctor; he had problems selecting the correct clothes to wear, was unable to do chores at home, got angry, had a short attention span, could not write or understand what he read, and other issues. He did poorly on the evaluation and was unable to draw a clock and tell time. He was diagnosed as being moderate to severely dysfunctional and had moderate dementia.

Ray was still able to drive his tractor and mow the fields as long as I rode along on the tractor to keep him focused on his task. He was still able to get exercise walking the dogs although he could not remember their names all the time.

However, about this time, I increasingly had to keep an eye on him because he started to wander off. He wanted to go back to his childhood home in Perryville, about 83 miles away. So I could locate him when he wandered off, I ordered a watch with a GPS service contract. The problem was he kept breaking the watch band and could not wear it. I prepaid for this service for a year without the benefit of its use. From here Ray moved to the next stage when *Dementia, The Monster Within,* is gaining strength and ready to cause major havoc in the person's brain.

From 2016 to 2018, Ray was at Stage Six (Severe cognitive decline). At this stage, some people would have moved their loved ones to a nursing home, but I could not afford it. I kept Ray at home despite the tremendous challenges in caring for him. This stage generally, lasts for four years, but Ray was only in this stage for two years. *The Monster Within* was continuing to rise and gain strength. In the summertime of 2016, Ray started to pick at his skin and developed sores. This is a key symptom that he was entering stage six. He picked at himself for about a year and a half and then quit.

So I could do my chores at the barn, I would leave Ray in the house but he left the house more and more often. A couple of times, he went through an atrium basement window to follow me down to the barn. Because he left the window open, the three dogs escaped. It took me an hour to catch the dogs and get everyone including Ray back in the house. I could not find any key locks for the vinyl basement windows so I had to find ways to block the windows. After the second time Ray climbed out that window, I put a table in front of the window and a heavy picnic table to hold it in place. The two other basement windows had plants in front of them and Ray could not figure out how to get around them to get to the windows. He continued to wander off, but did stay close to the house.

Eventually he increased his travels longer distances still wanting to return to his childhood home in Perryville. I would leave the house to work at the barn and return to the house and find him gone. I found him quickly most of the time by figuring out how far he could have traveled based on when I left the house, except twice.

I was working down at the barn taking care of the horses and he took off. I drove the roads, searching for him, but did not find him. I called the police who dispatched the Meramec Ambulance District EMT. They did find him, about a half mile from their station in Gray Summit, 15 miles away, and brought him home. The next time he took off he walked about 12 miles on a curvy and hilly road to the gas station in Cedar Hill. A gas station customer was a friend of Ray's brother and saw the family resemblance. He realized that Ray had cognitive issues, was lost and needed help. Fortunately when he asked Ray his name he did remember and the customer took him to his brothers' house who brought him back home.

Meanwhile, Ray's sister-in-law called me to say that Ray was located and that his brother was bringing him home. She said "Either Ray or the farm" meaning that she did not want her husband, Ray's brother, to be bothered again looking for Ray. I told her I would not get rid of the farm. I would find a way to successfully manage the farm and take care of Ray. She was not happy with my answer. I knew then that I would not receive much help for Ray's care from his relatives.

For Ray's own well-being, I did my best to involve family in his care. Ray always wanted to see his family. I did take Ray to visit at his brother's house twice in 2016 so he could watch him for me, but not for very long. They did not lock the doors to keep him in so I was always afraid that he would wander off. One time his brother and a friend did take him to a ballgame for his birthday, which Ray loved.

I also invited his relatives over for Christmas dinner with the last one being in 2018. I took Ray to see relatives at a couple of weddings, Thanksgiving dinners, his nephew's birthday party, and to visit relatives when they were in the hospital. Most of the time, I had to set up some type of event to get his relatives to visit him. Ray's brothers did help me twice (placing batteries in the diesel truck and adding wood panels in a barn).

Chapter 5: Escalating Anger

I was beginning to realize I would not receive much help for his care from friends and family because of his noticeable anger and personality changes. I was grateful to receive some help from another sister-in-law when she watched him for eight days in January 2016 so I could volunteer for the day at the Botanical Garden. On another occasion in 2017 a nice niece agreed to take him overnight at her home so I could volunteer at the Botanical Garden. Ray did wander off, and she was unable to follow him due to her injuries from an auto accident. However, she was able to send her grandnephew to follow him until I arrived. I had to miss another volunteer work day to retrieve him. Those were the only times I had any other help from any relative.

Another time that Ray wandered off, was at my sister's house for Christmas dinner. I was talking to my sister and not paying attention to him and he just walked off. We found him but left early due to his moodiness. Every situation is different and I learned to be flexible in dealing with his illness. By the next year, 2018, Ray was prescribed antipsychotic medications to control his violent behavior and now hallucinations. This also seemed to curb his wandering tendencies and Christmas Dinner 2018 at my sister's house he did not wander off. His behavior was also good at my dad's funeral in 2018 due to the medication.

About this time, I also had to stop him from driving the tractor because he could not shift the gears. This was one more skill he had lost to dementia. Ray still wanted to do the work but could not which made him very frustrated and angry. I am so glad that he had taught me how to drive the tractor before his health deteriorated. For a while I was able to let him ride on the back of the tractor so he could "help" and be with me. As the dementia progressed, I now had to mow the fields, myself. So he would not wander, I locked him in the house. He was growing angrier, but somehow I was still able to get work done that needed my attention.

After all those frightening wandering off adventures, I installed deadbolt locks on the doors and key locks on the windows to keep him in the house. One time, he removed a window lock, jumped down a story and a half without shoes and walked down to the barn to see me. To prevent this happening again I added a new keyed lock to that window. I also removed his shoes so it would be harder to walk off.

Once I started preventing him from wandering off, he got angrier and wanted to go back to his childhood home of Perryville. He would get his clothes out of the closet and try to take them with him on his trips. I retrieved them, put them back in the closet, and tried to distract him from his wandering episodes. He continued to try to take his clothes out until 2018 when realized that if I shut the closet door it prevented him from removing them. It seemed that if he could not see them, he would not remove them. This did not work all the time, but over time he stopped this behavior. I also stored his clothes in other places to keep him from taking them out. I learned to think of creative ways to handle new situations that arose.

In order to give Ray something to do, I bought a swing set for him and located it in the garage. I let him go to the garage to swing before dinner, but without his shoes so that he did not walk off. One time he did walk off without his shoes, but I followed him trying to get him to return. He got angry so I had a neighbor pick him up and take him to his house for change of pace. After some time for him to calm down, I returned to the neighbors and brought him home.

Every day he was getting more agitated and his anger was escalating. The length of time he was angry increased from a half an hour at time to two hours or more. Initially, he would only be angry couple days a month, but it escalated to maybe five or six days a week. In addition, he was beginning to hallucinate more (see images and hear sounds that were not there).

There were times I had to run away from him to avoid being injured. We had a center wall between the living room and the kitchen. I ran around the wall to get away from him. After a while he got tired of chasing me around and quit. Next, Ray started throwing things at me. Sometimes I had to jump on him to remove items (e.g. fireplace poker, kitchen utensils, books, family album, floor registers) that he could throw at me. He would get his nutrient drink from the refrigerator and throw it at me. He moved sofas, tables and threw chairs or coffee tables at me. Often, I had to leave the house and lock the doors behind me so he could not get out.

He banged on doors and broke door knobs with the floor registers or other items that I did not remove in time. I had to replace at least 12 door locks throughout the house that he broke. These episodes of anger and violence were extremely frightening and nerve racking. I sometimes ran to the basement and he chased after me. I outsmarted him by hiding in the darkest parts of the basement to prevent him from doing bodily harm to me. I was familiar with anger issues from my alcoholic dad; ranting, raving, and fighting with my mom during my adolescence. Compared to Ray's anger that was a "walk in the park". Ray's anger was just unbelievably unnerving, dangerous, unpredictable, and sometimes beyond words to describe.

Even the dogs (three big and one little dog) were afraid and ran away from him. I did not have time to keep the dogs separate, so they were stuck with him. He never did hurt them, but he chased them around. I often called my brother, Kevin, to give me comfort and assurance during these stressful events. Caregivers in these situations need someone they can trust to express their feelings and frustrations.

During another episode, he was angry because I left the house to go to the barn for something. When he saw me coming back to the house he started beating on the window. Because I was not quick enough to stop him, he broke the window. I quickly came in to see if he had hurt himself, which he did not. Then, he attacked me so I fought him off and went into the greenhouse. He kept banging on the greenhouse door so to prevent him from breaking that door's windows, I let him into the greenhouse with me. He hit me in the face and I fought him off and he finally left the greenhouse. He was walking off again and I taunted him back into the house so I could lock him inside. I had to be fast on my feet to get away from him and not be attacked again. I locked the doors and got back outside without him. I went out the garage so that he could not try to break anymore glass. One hour later, once he was calm, I reentered the house and everything was fine.

Ray gave me several minor injuries. He bruised my hand and hit me in the face twice. He tried to choke me several times, but I always managed to get away. In 2018 he threw a chair at me and did chip a small bone in my right hand. It healed with no lasting damage. I had to outsmart him and be versatile in my dealings with him. I still do not know how I coped with this violence for two years. His violence was like a wildfire that started with small embers and grew over time to burn several acres. The emotional toll it takes on a person is unbelievable.

Chapter 6: Finding Solutions

In June 2018, Ray's anger issues had escalated so much I had to do something. I learned of a Tuesday informational meeting at Barnes Hospital on palliative caregiving. From this, I discovered that there are behavioral centers that provide assistance in dealing with anger, violence, and mental illness. Also, I learned that Mercy Hospital had a Behavioral Center and that my insurance covered most of the expenses.

Ray had another one of his anger episodes on Friday that same week and that was the breaking point. He removed a light switch cover and stuck a sliver of wood from a cabinet door he broke into the switch. The switch burned but the breaker was tripped, preventing a fire. I repaired the switch but was afraid he would cause a fire in the house so I said "this is it!" I took him to the Mercy Behavioral Center the next day. He was upset when I left him there, but they were able to handle his moodiness. He was evaluated by a psychologist and prescribed anti-psychotic medications to manage his violence and hallucinations. He did cause a scene the next day and it took six guys to restrain him to give him an additional dose. He was released six days later on Thursday with these new medications to help manage his behavior.

Of course, I needed to look for my own psychologist to help me deal with Ray's behavior, which I found on Mercy Hospital's website. Mercy Behavioral Center also gave me a name of a great organization called Home Solutions. It is an organization that provides a ten week evaluation of your home care needs, trains the family caregiver, and supplies equipment. Home Solutions services are partially funded by Medicare.

Another source of assistance was the Alzheimer's Association. They provided me with some monies for a GPS tracking watch for Ray. As mentioned above the watch did not work out so well because Ray kept breaking it. The Alzheimer's Association has a wealth of information on dementia, which describes the types, and stages (early, middle, and late) of dementia.[3] They described the progression of the disease, how caregivers can prevent the person from becoming reactionary and what to do if the person is agitated.

I contacted Home Solutions and obtained an amazing amount of information. Home Solutions provided ten visits from July to October of 2018 to evaluate Ray's condition and provide recommendations. Home Solutions explained what dementia is, what the stages are, how it affects the person and that this disease is terminal. They teach you how to deal with the dementia patient by staying calm, limiting your conversation and using minimal directions for a task. Additionally, they made suggestions on activities for Ray, how to deal with the anger, how to prioritize needs, and to deal with disappointments and other obstacles.

They also mentioned that music had a tremendous calming effect on dementia patients. They provided headphones so Ray could always listen to music, but he did not like wearing them. He used them a little bit, but mostly listened to the radio that I placed in the living room for him. Every person is different and what works for one, may not work for someone else. As a caregiver, it is your role to find alternatives that work.

In October 2018, the Home Solutions occupational therapist, stated that she believed Ray was close to entering Stage Seven, the last stage (Very severe cognitive decline).

To help me manage this next stage of Ray's disease, Home Solutions provided safety items (e.g. slip proof treads, risers for the couch). In addition, they demonstrated equipment to assist Ray in the bathroom, which included a commode seat to provide support while using the toilet, a chair for the shower and grab bars. They then directed me to another organization called Aging Ahead who could provide the equipment I needed.

Aging Ahead obtains grants to provide money for caregivers to revamp the house for the dementia patient (e.g. stair rails, stairs, gates, and ramps), buy safety items for the bathroom, provide a grant for six hours a week of respite for the caregiver, and other programs. I obtained a commode seat, a chair for the shower and some grab bars through this organization. I also obtained six hours of respite care (Help At Home) every week until Ray died.

Home Solutions also introduced me to Project Lifesaver Program which is funded by the High Ridge Fire Department. This program provides, at no charge, a radio tracking device to find dementia and/or autistic patients that wander off. This program is being expanded to include all of Jefferson County residents. This is a low-cost method (no internet cost) to track people that have wandered off. They attached the tracker on an ankle and it is very hard to remove. Ray did manage to remove it a couple of times, but I was able to put it back on him. He was not able to wander off due to the locked doors, no shoes and eventually his desire to leave lessened. He was now walking mostly in the house and not outside very much. If he walked outside, I was with him. At this point, I was also helping Ray take a shower and dressing him.

Chapter 7: Preparing for Hospice

From 2018 to 2020, Ray entered Stage Seven, (Very severe cognitive decline) which generally lasts for two years. *The Monster Within* is in the final stage of destruction. Ray had crossed over. In about a six month period (November 2018 to May 2019) he started having urinary and fecal incontinence, his speech was limited to a few words, and he was having trouble getting up and down. The violence was less due, to the increased dosage of anti-psychotic medications and the drop in his energy level. He had forgotten who I was a few times, gave me blank stares, laughed at everything, even at sad events, clapped his hands for no reason, and was hallucinating more.

Ray was also not eating as much, sleeping more, but still occasionally had sundowner's syndrome anger manifestations. Sundowner's Syndrome is when dementia patients are more agitated and have more anger episodes, generally, after 3:00 p.m. Ray differed and had problems all the time, not just after 3:00 p.m.

I did manage to hire a caregiver in January 2018 to watch Ray while I volunteered at the Botanical Gardens and a few other days that I needed help. I also had a very nice neighbor watch him for me a couple of times. It was extremely hard to find someone to watch him at a reasonable price. I had to cobble together a small network of help from family, friends, and neighbors.

Several times I asked his favorite brother to come over and visit Ray, but he always had some excuse. Ray constantly asked me to call or ask his family to visit him throughout his illness. He was extremely sad and disappointed that they did not visit. Sometimes he would hallucinate and say his favorite brother was there when he was not. Family is very important at these times. It is sad for the patient to not be with family at a time in their lives when they are lonely, afraid, bored and emotional support is needed the most. This lack of family visits went on until the last week of Ray's life.

Ray's occupational therapist taught me what symptoms to look for as Ray's disease progressed; I suspected he was ready for hospice care in March of 2019. To qualify for the Medicare hospice program, the patient must be certified by the doctor and the hospice medical director as terminally ill and probably have less than six months to live.[4]

Chapter 8: Hospice Care

I contacted Ray's medical team to see if it was time to place Ray on hospice and yes, was the reply. He was put on hospice March 30, 2019. To my relief, hospice is 100% paid by Medicare. The hospice team was supervised by a physician and consisted of a nurse, nurse's aide, chaplain, and social worker that visited Ray weekly or biweekly. They provided family support, comfort to the terminally ill and medications and supplies (e.g. incontinent briefs, bed pads, razors for shaving). Throughout this stage they continually evaluated Ray's condition to ensure comfort until the end of his life.

As a part of the hospice program, the caregiver can request and be granted Medicare approved respite time off from caring for the patient. In May and June 2019, I had my first respite time away from Ray for six days and five nights. This is not monthly, just sporadically, whenever needed and if the time is approved by Medicare. Respite consisted of placing Ray in an approved facility, such as a nursing home for that time. The respite program was beneficial but some nursing homes lose patients clothes even if they are labeled. I had to replace some of Ray's clothes at an expense of over $400 over time.

The hospice program also provided volunteers to watch him, which did not work out very well for me. The volunteers are not adequately trained to deal with more difficult situations such as I encountered. As previously stated, Ray was an extremely, challenging person to deal with and sometimes I lost my temper (I am human).

One time when the volunteer was present, I lost my temper and yelled at Ray. She did not understand why I was mad at him and did not think it was justified. She decided not to volunteer for me anymore. The second volunteer wanted me to always stay close by. I live on a farm with horses that I care for, in addition to caring for Ray. The stables are not close to the house. I was feeding the horses at the barn and just five minutes delayed getting back to the house and she freaked out. She thought something had happened and she called the hospice volunteer coordinator. I told her that I was, simply down at the barn feeding the horses and was here, not to worry.

This volunteer got upset a second time because I was seven minutes late answering the door. I happened to be struggling to get Ray showered and dressed after an incontinence episode. She went into the same frenzy as before. I was emotional because of the battle with Ray and asked that she give me more time to get to the door and not to get so upset. She thought I was yelling at her although I even apologized for my emotional state.

She refused to volunteer for me anymore and spoke to the nurse in charge who gave me a not so nice phone call. The nurse stated that I had treated the two volunteers poorly and informed me that I would not receive any more volunteers. From my viewpoint, the volunteers were not qualified to handle situations as difficult as mine and needed a lot more training/experience. They also needed more information on what situations they will encounter such as sensitivity training for the caregivers needs. Like I said, caregiving is not "a walk in the park" and is extremely emotional and draining.

Since Ray was on hospice, he had a special DNR (do not resituate) medical instruction. This means that if Ray had an emergency, then a hospice team member is called, instead of an ambulance. CPR will not be performed. However, if he had a minor non-life threatening, illness a hospice nurse would provide whatever care is required to make him comfortable. The hospice program provides comprehensive medical care, with no more trips required to the doctor. If he falls and injures himself, then the hospice team will evaluate and if required arrange transport to the hospital.

By October 2019, Ray was progressively getting more disabled. He was sleeping more, had a lot of trouble getting up, was not walking as much, skipped a meal or two occasionally, talked very little but fortunately, because of his lack of energy, he was less angry. Because of his size and unwillingness to cooperate, I was having trouble getting him to the car to take him to get his hair cut or see the dentist.

Ray was regularly combative when a particular nurse's aide gave him a shower. Fortunately, we were able to change to a different aide and he was more willing to take a shower. Some days he still refused to cooperate so, the hospice organization would provide two nurse aides to help.

I received more respite time in September and October 2019 when Ray was allowed a stay in a nursing home. Because he had to be heavily sedated in the nursing home to keep him calm and not violent, he lost his ability to walk very well. Back at home, it took a week and a half for him to recover from the Ativan, prescribed to treat anxiety during his nursing home respite stays.

When he came home from the nursing home, I had major problems moving him. The first day he was back I struggled, but managed by myself to get him from the couch to the kitchen chair to eat and back to the couch. He was 6′2″ weighing about 165 lbs. and I was 5′2″ weighing 123 lbs. It was not easy, but I was inventive. Since he could not walk, I helped him crawl or get up with my help and used a dog mattress for him to rest upon until we could get to the couch.

To help with mobility, I ordered a hospital bed and a wheelchair for Ray. The hospital bed had side rails and could be raised or lowered with a jointed mattress base so that the head may also be adjusted. In addition they provided a table and a large floor mat to cushion any falls. Unfortunately, this bed did not have an overhead grab bar or the two foot bed extension for my tall husband. After Ray had died I found out from an employee of the rental company that you can order these additional items. Also, I learned from the hospice nurse I could have ordered a hoist to lift him up from the bed. However, a two to three person team is required to move the hoist, which was not practical for my situation.

In November 2019, after he recovered from his nursing home respite, Ray was still walking fine, but began to decline in other ways physically. He was becoming more incontinent and was extremely messy to clean up and it only got worse. Friday afternoons a caregiver stayed with Ray while I ran errands. Every time I left, Ray would become very anxious and walk in circles around the center wall between the living room and the kitchen, upsetting the caregiver.

In anticipation of Ray needing more care, a few of my errand trips, were to evaluate and look for nursing homes to place Ray in come January 2020. When Ray could not get up anymore I figured that insurance would cover placing him in a nursing home. Initially, the insurance company said that they cover all types of hospice care in a nursing home, but I learned that is not correct. They do not cover hospice care in a nursing home for patients with dementia as the primary disease. If Ray required temporary rehabilitative skilled nursing care for wounds, dialysis, rehab therapy, blood transfusions, or other treatments, he could be admitted into a nursing home for up to 210 days. This would have been covered 100% by his insurance. Unfortunately, insurance did not cover Ray's care in a nursing home because he did not require skilled nursing attention.

Generally patients are in the hospice program for six months or less unless they have not passed away. But if the patient continues to decline they can continue on hospice until they die. Since Ray did not improve he continued on hospice for a total of 11 months.

I had many long discussions with nursing homes, insurance agents and skilled nurses on Medicare coverage. Medicare Guidelines states, **"No, custodial or long term care for dementia patients"** where the help is really needed. I finally realized that with no insurance coverage, I could not afford to place him in a nursing home. I continued to struggle with Ray's care and call in favors of people to help me when they could. I did not obtain any paid nursing help in the home due to the cost ($25 an hour or more) and Ray needed 24 hour care.

Chapter 9: Physical Decline and Passing

In December 2019, I noticed Ray was starting to have stomach pain and loss of appetite. I thought it was due to the dementia progression. He was walking less and having more trouble getting to his feet; he needed more assistance and I was having more difficulty providing it.

I had scheduled respite care at a different nursing home this time. However, because of a big snowstorm we moved the date for respite back so I could shovel our long driveway. Ray was just fine in the nursing home for two days, then all hell broke loose. He had eaten something that apparently irritated his stomach and when the nurses' aides took him for a shower he fought them. He then struck two nurses so they called me to take him and not to ever return.

Hospice suggested moving him to a behavioral center to get his anger issues resolved. They transported him to the Sullivan Hospital Emergency Room to be checked out before being transported to the behavioral center. However, we learned there was not a bed available in the behavioral center. In the Emergency Room, he was extremely agitated and angry. He tried to punch anyone that touched him. They finally gave him Ativan, which calmed him down so that they could diagnose him. He was running a fever of 103 and was in extreme pain so they tested for a gallbladder disease which was positive. Finally late that evening he was admitted to the hospital.

While he was in the hospital he also struck a nurse as well. His relatives did come and visit him a couple of the days he was in the hospital. He was in the hospital for four days and was released on Christmas Eve 2019 without going to a behavioral center so his new medications could be adjusted.

I brought him home Christmas Eve and put him on a low-fat diet to reduce the gallbladder pain. He was unable to walk very much at all now. I was barely able to get him in the house and into bed. He was starting to be bedbound. I called my one special girlfriend to come out Christmas Day and help change him. We did fine with the change, but it was getting harder because he could not help. The next day he was placed back on hospice and the nurse practitioner helped me change him. He did get up by himself and walk to the couch in the living room to sleep. Because of his incontinence, I did not want him sleeping on the couch but decided to wait and move him back to bed the next day. I still had to pick my battles.

The next day Ray was still on the couch and I wanted him back in bed. Since he was difficult to move, I decided to push him off the couch onto the floor and had him crawl to the bed. Then, I had him lean on the lowered bed and I swung his lower body up onto the bed. I struggled with his care throughout the holidays and into January. He was getting more and more unable to help me and was eating less. One time I forgot about his special diet and gave him some salmon which affected his gallbladder. He did not spike a fever, but it caused him pain. I was allowed to give him morphine to relieve pain now that he was on hospice.

The first week in January 2020 I did get more neighbors to help me change him. On Monday, I did not have any help to change him so I had to do it myself. Ray did not like the nurse's method of turning him in bed from one side to another side to clean and change the bed linens. He fought every part of that process.

I did not want to go through that struggle and I was physically unable to turn him by myself. So, I developed my own creative method. I had him sit up in bed and I lowered the bed to the lowest setting. I laid a large mat for falls on the floor in front of him. I told him that I was going to push him out of bed down about six inches onto a floor mat onto all fours. He agreed with this plan and I was able to change his pants, and clean him and the bed. To get him back in bed, I had him crawl back to the bed and lay over the bed. I was able again to swing him up on the clean bed and get him comfortable. I did the process as quickly and safely as possible. This turned out to be the best way to clean and change him.

The second week in January was his last week of life. He ate less and less, slept more and stayed in bed. He did not want to get up into the wheelchair except for me to change him. His energy level was falling. I had a neighbor help change him on Monday and the next day the nurses changed him without a fight, which was very unusual. He was eating less and not drinking very much so I was able to skip a day to clean him up.

That Thursday I had my sister and her husband come out and help me. It was a great relief to have this help. The process went ok and they stated how frail, skinny and weak he had become. That Friday, three days before his death, he was catheterized by the hospice nurse. That was also the last day he ate anything and he was unable to take his normal meds anymore. He was on morphine and Ativan only.

He started to go in and out of a coma. I want to note that he never did have any swallowing issues that most patients have during their final stage of life. They also lose the ability to smile and sit up in bed. Ray could sit up but not smile, due to his comatose state. The hospice nurse mentioned several times during our conversations that Ray will probably go quickly once he quits walking. He did not linger long in the bedridden stage before death which, even, surprised the nurse.

I was finally able to get his two brothers and their wives over to visit him on the Saturday before he died. He did wake up enough to know that they were there for a few minutes. They were saying to me that they thought he could live a lot longer. I told them that he was in and out of a coma and was about to die. They also asked why there were no fluid tubes in his arms and where were the nurses. They did not understand that hospice is to just keep the terminally ill patient comfortable and that life support treatments are not used.

The hospice nurse did show up to check on him that Saturday morning during Ray's relative's visit. She explained to them that he was on hospice and that uncomfortable life support measures are not used when someone is about to die. She explained that our goal was to provide comfort and prevent pain while he dies, not to stop or prolong the process. She said to call if needed. Also, she provided directions to dispense more morphine if his pain increased. My in-laws were satisfied with her explanation concerning hospice. They left after the visit never to see him alive again.

While Ray's relatives were visiting we had a long discussion about Medicaid and Medicare. I cleared up a lot of their misunderstandings about the Medicaid program eligibility and property ownership requirements.

Medicaid is a program for people with no financial resources. However, more and more middle income people are considering using Medicaid to cover the high costs of long term care. Ray's relatives did not realize the strict qualifications for Medicaid. Every state is different. In Missouri, as of August 20, 2020, in my situation, we were limited to an income of about $1370 per month to be eligible for Medicaid.[5]

Once you apply for Medicaid, you are required to spend down your savings to a certain level. Many people to prepare for care in later life, consider gifting their money or property to a family member. Medicaid does not allow the patient to hide or transfer their funds and will "look back" three years from the date applied for Medicaid to locate financial resources. The spouse caregiver can usually keep the house and their portion of monies however, with the death of the remaining spouse or when the property is sold, Medicaid must recover the cost of the care provided.

Ray continued to stay in a coma all day on Sunday and briefly woke up saying "help".

He needed more morphine to keep him comfortable. His organs were shutting down and he was in pain. I checked on him at 11:30 p.m. and he was still breathing. I went to bed and woke up at 3:00 a.m. on Monday and found him deceased. *The Monster Within* had won. I called the nurse and she came over to pronounce him dead. She also called the funeral home and we cleaned him up for the funeral home to take his body.

I called his niece and nephew and asked the nephew to go with me to the funeral home to identify the body and make the arrangements. Yes, I had to view his body that went from ghostly at home to ghastly at the funeral home after a few hours of decomposition.

To end his story, Ray was cremated and about two weeks later we had a memorial service celebrating his life, not his death. It was a well-attended beautiful service and the hospice chaplain gave a nice send off. Several people presented their humorous experiences with Ray

during his lifetime.   He would have been
impressed with such a nice memorial.

Chapter 10: Some Recommendations

Missouri does not have a very good support system for caring for dementia or elderly loved ones. All forms of dementia are on the rise as baby boomers age. We will need more facilities, support staff, medications, nurses, doctors and caregivers to manage this increase in care. Although we spend our lives paying our tax dollars for Medicare, our health care system does not provide the benefits really needed. As more middle income taxpayers wrestle with caring for loved ones, we need to act now, not later.

The primary alternative most agencies recommend to caregivers is extremely, costly nursing homes that charge a fortune to provide for loved ones. Yes, there is a place for nursing homes, but how can some afford it. If I had placed Ray in a nursing home, four years ago, and not kept him at home, I would have had to shell out well over $350,000 to pay for his care. Caregivers should not have to decide between caring for their loved ones and losing their homes and life savings.

Medicare needs reform. The first issue that needs reform is the patient protection law. The law requires the social worker (wardens of the state) to notify the police if abuse and/or neglect has been observed. These laws that protect the patient can also imprison the caregivers who provide care 24/7. For example, if the caregivers must leave the loved ones at home for a short time to get medications or groceries, and someone else is not present, then they can be fined or jailed for neglect and abuse. This is an example of "damned if you do and damned if you don't". How is this in the best interest of the patient to lose the only caregiver to jail and/or fines? Caregivers need to be let out of their home prison. Caregivers require more time to do errands and for themselves after struggling to take care of their dementia patient nonstop.

A second issue that needs to be addressed is education for the police on dementia and understanding how to handle certain situations. When Ray wandered off, and I contacted the police for help, they treated me like I had done something wrong. The officer wanted to talk to Ray and kept putting me off. Ray was confused but stated to the officer that he was fine so the officer left without understanding all aspects of the situation. The police need training on sensitivity for all parties and to understand that the behaviors of people with dementia ranges from confusion, to anger and violence.

Third, Medicare needs to provide subsided paid labor to help caregivers through this disease. Paying for additional caregiver help is expensive and relying on friends and family to help is not always possible. Some family members are reluctant to help and the responsibility usually falls on just one principal caregiver often with limited resources. Caregivers are in a home prison, taking care of our loved ones. Where is the justice in this! Why do we have to wear shackles to provide the needed care?

Because of my experience as a caregiver, I have some suggestions on what services need to be covered to provide more caregiver assistance. Subsidize day care centers through grants or Medicare funds and charge only a nominal fee ($30) instead of over $100 a day. Nursing homes should be subsidized, and charge $1,000 to $2,000 a month instead of $5,500 to $10,000 and up. Home health care should be subsidized by Medicare to reduce the cost to the caregiver from $25 to $30 an hour to $10 an hour (eight hours or less is currently $200 a day). Medicare also should provide caregivers with funds to cover more time (15 hours a week) for respite and custodial care. In the long run, it would save money by keeping the caregiver healthier from battling the burden of caregiving.

Lastly, I was helped by several private organizations, such as Aging Ahead, who obtained grants to help me pay private home care organizations. It would be great if more of these private organizations could share their skills through some sort of clearing house. Caregivers need a way to find real resources to help provide care. I was fortunate to just stumble upon the real resource (the resources that Aging Ahead provided) that provided some relief to my financial and caregiving dilemmas.

It will take billions of dollars to pay for these services. Congress and the powers to be need to consider how to provide the support that is required. It's estimated that beginning in 2024, Medicare will not have enough money to pay for all of the expected hospital expenses. Reform is needed to help families and caregivers. Reform proposals have been discussed for years. The first category of reform would layer changes to Medicare on top of its current structure, in which the government sets the terms of coverage and the prices for health services. The second approach to Medicare reform would instead transform Medicare into a marketplace of regulated, private health plans with government-provided subsidies for the premiums.[6]

Missouri has one of the lowest funded Medicaid programs in the country. Something needs to be done to provide adequate assistance to needy families caring for loved ones.

I challenge congressmen, lobbyists, caregivers and any others concerned about people with dementia to come up with help now, not later. The federal government and states should step up and provide more aid. *The Monster Within* is in dementia as well as our medical system. We need reform.

I have a final challenge to the families that have loved ones with dementia. Caregivers need help from all family members. Do not turn your back on the people that need you the most while they are ill. Family needs to be there for the dementia patient and not ignore the need for emotional support. Family members provide so much comfort when they visit in person since the patient can see them and know that they care. They do not even need to talk to the patient. This is a simple gift of time and comfort that an ill person appreciates very much. Ray constantly asked for his favorite brother to be there for him, but that did not always happen, and he was extremely sad and heartbroken. That was one more obstacle that Ray had to face, not feeling loved by his family members because they did not understand. Ray felt abandoned.

I hope this book gives everyone a glimpse into what happens when a person gets dementia. I hope Ray's story will enlighten and inform. I have shared information on what to expect, the **deficiencies** of our medical system, the disease progression and how the person is affected. Yes, Ray went through hell and I had lot of challenges with his care. Not everyone will be so violent. Before this disease, he was a wonderful person, helping anyone that asked him to do projects, adventurous, loved travel, a hard worker, and a fun-loving guy. *The Monster Within* beat Ray, but through research and education we can win for others. I hope Ray will not be just a statistic, but a link to conquer this disease. We need funding for the medical system to provide more support to the caregiver and the patient.

After going through several years of caring for Ray with all the freedom restrictions placed on me, now we are confronted with the covid-19 pandemic restrictions. I have been prepared by staying at home to care for Ray for three years; one year is nothing. I am thankful that Ray died when he did, before the shutdowns, so that I could have people at the memorial service to honor him. It is so hard now for people not to be able to be with their dying loved ones and unable to attend their funerals. Life is tough, just do not lose hope and give up even in the worst of times. Be brave, listen to science, not <u>politics,</u> and we will get through this pandemic also.

Hospice also offers bereavement services for the caregivers and family. Due to the pandemic restrictions, I have not been able participate any social events, except by phone. This is just another challenge to get through. We should all strive to conquer *The Monster Within* and other challenges in our lives. After this pandemic is over, visit your neighbors, family, friends, and live life again. Life is too precious not to enjoy it to the fullest.

References

[1] 1984 by Barry Weisberg, M.D. All rights reserved. Weisberg. Functional Assessment Staging (FAST). Psychopharmacology Bulletin. 1988:24: 653-659.

[2] 'donepezil - oral, Aricept', *MedicineNet, Inc*, San Clemente, Calif., https://www.medicinenet.com/donepezil-oral/article.htm, (accessed 2 March 2021)

[3] Alzheimer's Association, St. Louis Chapter's, Basic Dementia Care Guide, 1999, revised 2011 and 2015.

[4] 'Hospice care', *Medicare.gov*, https://www.medicare.gov/coverage/hospice-care, (accessed 3 March 2021)

[5] 'Missouri Medicaid / MO HealthNet Income & Asset Limits for Nursing Homes & In-Home Long Term Care', *MedicaidPlanningAssistance.org*, American Council on Aging, December 15, 2020, https://www.medicaidplanningassistance.org/medicaid-eligibility-missouri/, (accessed 28 March 2021)

[6] Daniel P. Kessler, 'Real Medicare Reform', National Affairs, Fall 2012, https://www.nationalaffairs.com/publications/detail/real-medicare-reform, (accessed 1 March 2021)